Table of Contents

Multiple sclerosis (or MS) is an autoimmune disease that affects the central nervous system. MS affects 2.5 million people worldwide and around 400,000 people in the United States.

What are the symptoms of MS and how is it diagnosed? MS symptoms affect each person differently. They can include weakness, numbness, cognitive changes and blurred vision. Currently there is no single test that is used for diagnosing multiple sclerosis, so multiple tests will often need to be performed. Doctors will usually diagnose MS based on a patient's symptoms, a physical examination and results from magnetic resonance imaging tests (MRI).

What age does multiple sclerosis start? MS can develop at any age and affects women more often than men. The disorder is most commonly diagnosed between ages 20 and 40, but can be seen in both younger and older people.

Because it's not entirely known what causes MS, there is no "cure" for the condition. The good news is that there are multiple sclerosis natural treatments that often can cause a great improvement in symptoms, and, when combined with other approaches, might even be able to help reverse the condition.

Chapter one

What Is Multiple Sclerosis?

According to the National Multiple Sclerosis Society:

Multiple sclerosis (MS) is an unpredictable, often disabling disease of the central nervous system that disrupts the flow of information within the brain, and between the brain and body.

Multiple sclerosis refers to many (multiple) areas of tissue scarring (sclerosis) and damage. The main type of tissue that is damaged by MS is called myelin, the tissue that wraps around nerves and helps nerve fibers send chemical signals throughout the body.

When myelin is damaged it's called demyelination. Some of the earliest signs and symptoms of multiple sclerosis include changes in sense of touch, loss of strength in one arm or leg, tingling, burning and itching. When myelin is damaged, nerve signals reaching the eyes, brain and spinal cord slow down or stop. As MS worsens with time the brain can sometimes shrinks in size as more myelin and axons are destroyed, leading to decreased cognitive functioning and many other symptoms related to nervous system dysfunction.

Can you be born with multiple sclerosis? Most people who develop MS do so as young adults. It's not exactly known what causes all cases of MS, but experts believe that one common cause might be exposure to viruses early in life. Examples of two viruses that might trigger MS include herpesvirus and retrovirus. It's possible to start developing symptoms of MS early in life but not receive a diagnosis until years later when the condition has progressed.

Symptoms and Signs

MS symptoms include those that are sensory (resulting in problems with sensations) and related to motor control (muscle movements and coordination). The most common multiple sclerosis symptoms include:

- Vision changes including blurred or double vision. Some might experience partial blindness, dimmed vision, inability to see straight ahead (central vision loss) and uncoordinated movements of the eyes. Vision changes are due to increased inflammation of the optic nerves leading to the eyes (optic neuritis).

- Cognitive changes and mental impairment, including trouble thinking clearly, memory loss, poor judgement and inattention.
- Lack of coordination, clumsy movements and loss of balance.
- Numbness, tingling, reduced sense of touch.
- Sense of shock running down the neck and spinal cord, especially when moving the head/neck.
- Burning, itching or pain on the skin.
- Cramping, spasms and weakness in the arms or legs, tremors, trouble walking, and stiffness.
- Mood changes, including mood swings, depression or manic depression, inability to control emotions, increasing crying and inappropriate laughing.

- Sexual dysfunction, including lack of sensation in the genitals, trouble experiencing pleasure or orgasm and impotence.
- Dizziness and vertigo.
- Digestive symptoms including constipation, diarrhea/loss of control over bowel movements, and trouble controlling urination.
- Slowed, slurred and hesitant speech.
- Partial paralyzation and involuntary movements as the condition worsens.
- Dementia and mania as the condition worsens.

Relapses and Remission in Multiple Sclerosis Symptoms

MS symptoms can vary widely from person to person. It's common for MS symptoms to come and go, as many people experience alternating periods of remission and relapses (or flare-ups). This means that it's common for people with MS to feel relatively healthy for a period of time followed by a period of feeling ill as symptoms worsen.

There are several different types of multiple sclerosis that describe the severity of the disease and also the fluctuations between remission and flare-ups. The reason that remission and flare-ups occur is because the myelin surrounding nerves may be repaired, then damaged again, then repaired again, and so on. Remissions in MS symptoms can last for months or even years. The majority of people with MS — about 80 percent–85 percent — have relapsing-remitting MS.

Relapses of multiple sclerosis symptoms can be debilitating in some cases, but mild in others. Most of the time recovery from MS will only be short-lived and incomplete, as the condition tends to get worse with time. Some might have only a single ongoing symptom and go months or years without experiencing any others. A flare in symptoms can sometimes only happen one time, go away, and never return. For other people the symptoms are more usually intense and may become worse within weeks or months of them first beginning. This is called "primary progressive pattern." When MS remissions and flare-ups alternate it is called "secondary progressive pattern" or "progressive relapsing pattern."

Causes and Risk Factors

What does multiple sclerosis do to the body that causes the symptoms described above? As mentioned above, MS is caused by damage to the myelin sheath, the protective covering that surrounds nerve cells. Nerves are covered by tissue (myelin) that acts like insulation, much like the coating used to protect electric wires. The covering of nerves is needed to help conduct nerve impulses and therefore many bodily functions, such as muscle coordination and control over emotions.

The kind of nerve damage that is associated with MS is caused by factors including autoimmune responses, dysbiotic gut microbiota, and increased inflammation. In other words, MS is believed to be caused by the body's own immune cells attacking the nervous system. This damage can happen anywhere in the brain or spinal cord.

Although no specific causes of MS are known, some possible causes include:

Viruses and infections, such as herpesvirus or retrovirus.

Mold toxicity.

Toxic exposure and heavy metal posioning.

Vitamin D deficiency, especially during the early stages of life. It's been found that living near the equator/in a tropical climate, where vitamin D deficiency is less common due to more sunlight exposure, lowers someone's risk for MS substantially. People living in temperate climates where it is cooler and darker are more likely to be deficient in vitamin D and considered to be at an increased risk for developing MS.

Food allergies.

Immunizations.

Heredity, or family history of MS and similar conditions. It's estimated that about 5 percent of people with multiple sclerosis have a sibling who is also affected, and about 15 percent have a close relative with MS. It's been found that people with certain genetic markers (human leukocyte antigens) are at an increased risk for MS.

Hormonal imbalances.

High levels of emotional stress (this may not be the underlying cause but can trigger symptom flare-ups).

A poor diet that causes inflammation, poor gut health and nutrient deficiencies.

Other risk factors for multiple sclerosis include: Being between the ages of 20–40. Of the 400,000 people living in the U.S. that have MS, the majority are believed to be young adults under 40.

Being a woman.

Smoking cigarettes.

Childhood obesity. Some research shows that those with a high body mass index (BMI) before age 20 may be twice as likely to develop MS as those within a normal weight range.

Vitamin D deficiency during the first 15 years of life.

Some of the most common causes of a flare in MS symptoms include:

Having a fever, the flu, a virus or another illness that stresses the immune system.

Lack of sleep and increased stress.

Overexertion and dehydration.

Spending time in very hot temperatures or situations, such as being in a sauna, experiencing heat exhaustion or even taking very hot baths.

Hormonal fluctuations.

Natural Treatments

Conventional treatments for multiple sclerosis typically include use of corticosteroid drugs that help to suppress the immune system and limit autoimmune reactions. Steroids are used to stop the body from attacking its own cells and tissue, while other drugs might be used to treat specific symptoms such as weakness, tingling and blurred vision. Recently a number of "disease modifying drugs" have been developed that are given to patients with MS to help lengthen the time of remission periods and to lower the severity of flare-ups. These drugs don't work for every person and all types of MS, but can be very helpful for some.

Meanwhile, a promising clinical trial led by Dr. Richard Burt of Northwestern University that explores the potential benefits of stem cell therapy for multiple sclerosis is underway as of March 2018. The 110 patients participating either received a drug treatment or hematopoietic stem cell transplantation (HSCT). The clinical trial looks promising given that after one year of treatment only one relapse occurred among patients in the stem cell group compared with 39 relapses in the drug treatment. And, after about three years, the stem cell transplants had a 6 percent failure rate compared with a failure rate of 60 percent in the control (drug treatment) group.

The researchers note that stem cell therapy doesn't work for all cases of MS and it's not an easy process. First patients must undergo chemotherapy to destroy their "faulty" immune system. Then stem cells that help make blood through a process called hematopoiesis are removed from the patient's bone marrow and reinfused into the patient's bloodstream. These fresh stem cells, which are not affected by MS, rebuild the patient's immune system. Despite this challenging process, preliminary results demonstrate that this could be an effective treatment in the future.

Unfortunately, currently, even with treatment it's still common for MS to slowly worsen over time, sometimes leaving people disabled and unable to live on their own. However, the good news is that the lifespan of people living with multiple sclerosis is usually unaffected, unless the disorder becomes very severe. Below are examples of multiple sclerosis natural treatments that can also help manage symptoms and improve quality of life:

Nutrient-Dense Diet High in Healthy Fats

A 2015 report published in the journal ASN Neuro states:

Dietary factors and lifestyle may exacerbate or ameliorate MS symptoms by modulating the inflammatory status of the disease, both in relapsing-remitting MS and in primary-progressive MS. This is achieved by controlling both the metabolic and inflammatory pathways in the human cell and the composition of commensal gut microbiota.

No specific type of diet has been proven to prevent or cure multiple sclerosis. But there is some evidence that following a diet that's high in antioxidants and healthy fats can be one of several basic multiple sclerosis natural treatments that may help with symptom management. Experts believe that high-calorie, highly-processed "Western diets" may be a trigger for MS and other neurological disorders. MS is more prevalent in Western countries with the highest income (and also the greatest distance from the equator). Western diets are characterized by high amounts of salt, animal fat, factory-farm-raised red meat, sugar-sweetened drinks, fried food and low-fiber foods. To top it off, most people eating a Western diet are not getting enough physical exercise and potentially lacking sleep and time for relaxation too.

A study published in 2018 assessed the association between diet quality and the intake of particular foods with the severity of symptoms in multiple sclerosis patients. Participants in the study completed a dietary questionnaire that estimated the intake of red/processed meats, whole grains, added sugars, fruits, vegetables and legumes to construct a diet quality score based on the reported food groups. In addition to the food groups, the questionnaire also assessed whether an overall healthy lifestyle (healthy weight, diet, physical activity and smoking abstinence) is associated with symptom severity of MS. Out of the respondents, those with MS whose diet quality scores were in the highest percentile had lower levels of disability and depression. Those with an overall healthy lifestyle had lower chances of reporting severe fatigue, pain, depression or cognitive impairment. The study concludes that the healthier choices in diet and lifestyle contributed to a lighter burden of disability and symptoms associated with MS.

Fats are essential nutrients for forming and protecting the nerves' myelin sheath, while antioxidants help to reduce oxidative damage. Aim to eat a diet that is similar to the Mediterranean diet, which research shows helps to reduce inflammation, protect cognitive health, reduce cardiovascular mortality risk, and improve endothelial functions. Foods to include in a healthy multiple sclerosis diet are:

Unprocessed foods — Choose whole, organic, unprocessed foods as often as possible.

Coconut Oil — Coconut oil contains large amounts of medium chain fatty acids (MCFA) that support the brain and nervous system. Olive oil is another healthy source of fat that is associated with cognitive health.

Fresh fruits and vegetables — Aim for a variety of colors to provide antioxidants that can help prevent free radical damage and inflammation. Plant foods that provide sulforaphane (SFN) — an organosulfur compound that has potent anti-oxidant and anti-inflammatory activities — are some of the best foods for managing MS because they reduce inflammation, oxidative stress, demyelination and autoimmune responses. The best sources of sulforaphane are cruciferous vegetables such as Brussels sprouts, broccoli, cabbage, cauliflower, bok choy, kale and collards.

Foods high in polyphenols — For example, vegetables, whole grains, legumes, spices, herbs, fruits, wine, fruit juices, tea and coffee.

Foods high in lycopene and carotenoids — These include plant foods like tomatoes, carrots, watermelon, sweet potatoes, winter squash and grapefruit.

Omega-3 fats — The EPA/DHA fats found in wild-caught fish (and fish oil supplements) can help reduce inflammation. The best omega-3 foods include wild salmon, sardines, mackerel, trout and herring.

Prebiotics and probiotics — These are "beneficial bacteria" that help to restore or maintain a healthy symbiotic gut microbiota. Probiotic foods include fermented dairy products like yogurt or kefir (if dairy is tolerated well), cultured veggies and kombucha. Prebiotic foods include raw dandelion greens, raw garlic, raw leeks or onions, raw jicama, raw asparagus and under-ripe bananas.

Complex carbohydrates — Examples include ancient grains that are high in fiber such as millet and sorghum. Complex carbs may help with the growth of beneficial bacteria in the gut, helping to control inflammation.

Cabbage and bean sprouts — Foods high in lecithin may help strengthen the nerves.

Foods to avoid in order to help with MS recovery include:

Processed foods — Reduce your exposure to chemicals and toxins by avoiding any foods that are processed. Try to eat whole foods (foods that are only one ingredient) and check ingredient labels on packaged foods to avoid additives and chemicals. Avoid foods with lots of saturated fatty acids of animal origin, hydrogenated fatty acids, added sweeteners/artificial sweeteners, refined carbohydrates, lots of added salt, MSG, and cow's milk.

Gluten — Certain food allergies and sensitivities are known to make MS symptoms worse. People with MS may be more prone to having a gluten-intolerance. Gluten might make symptoms worse for some people with MS, which is why a gluten-free diet is recommended.

Dairy — Just like with gluten, people with MS may have a harder time digesting cow's milk. A dairy-free diet might be able to help manage symptoms and improve gut health, although it depends on the person.

Potential food allergens — Allergens may make MS symptoms worse by triggering autoimmune reactions, so carefully avoid any foods you might be allergic to.

Sugar — Too much sugar in the diet may disrupt immune responses and contribute to systemic inflammation and premature aging.

Alcohol — Above moderate levels, alcohol can increase inflammation and can create a toxic bodily environment.

Limit Exposure to Viruses and Infections

Below are steps you can take to practice good hygiene and prevent catching illnesses from those around you that can trigger a flare-up:

Wash your hands regularly, especially after going to the bathroom.

Avoid sharing personal items, such as towels or razors, that can carry bodily fluids.

Regularly wash all fabrics and linens using a natural antibacterial detergent. Wash all dirty clothes containing bodily fluids, towels and bedding, particularly after they come into contact with someone who has an infection.

Clean and disinfect all working surfaces thoroughly and regularly. Frequently disinfect shared items in your home or workplace using natural cleaning products.

Food workers should always wash their hands thoroughly to prevent foodborne illnesses from spreading.

If you go to a gym or exercise facility, make sure to clean equipment after use and shower once you leave.

- Exercise and Reduce Stress

When considering multiple sclerosis natural treatments, physical exercise is now a very common approach for MS patients as it has been shown to decrease the symptoms of chronic fatigue, help with stress management, improve coordination and prevent or slow the onset of disability. MS patients should practice mild physical exercise, such as brisk walking, swimming, light dancing, yoga, tai chi or light cycling. Working with a trainer in a rehabilitation center or program is also encouraged.

Some of the ways that exercise benefits MS include upregulating oxidative metabolism and downregulating biosynthetic pathways and inflammation. It helps to support energy balance, influences quality of life and may stimulate the production of anti-inflammatory cytokines. In animal studies, exercise has also been shown to stimulate brain mitochondrial activity, to improve neuroplasticity, improve moods and decrease anxiety.

Exercise is considered part of a "holistic treatment plan," which includes diet, exercise, therapy, stress management and social support. Controlling emotional and physical stress is important for reducing relapses and prolonging remission. Some activities that can help with stress management include yoga, deep breathing, meditation, massages, exercise, journaling, reading, support groups and prayer.

Prevent or Treat Vitamin D Deficiency

It is not exactly clear how vitamin D helps prevent multiple sclerosis, but it is known that deficiency in vitamin D can lower immune function and have an effect on neurological development. Studies have uncovered evidence suggesting that vitamin D deficiency during childhood may be most problematic. In animal studies it's been found that there's a "developmental stage-dependent efficiency of vitamin D to ameliorate neuroinflammation," pointing to the need to prevent low vitamin D levels during childhood and adolescence.

The best way to make enough vitamin D on your own is to expose your bare skin to sunlight everyday, if possible, for about 15 minutes. If you live in a place where it's very dark and cold, or during the winter, then you can supplement with vitamin D3 (5,000 IU daily) to help modulate the immune system and support your brain and nervous system.

Take Helpful Supplements

Below are some supplements that can be used as multiple sclerosis natural treatments to help support the immune system and aid in preventing MS symptoms such as fatigue and weakness:

Fish oil (2,000 milligrams daily) — Fish oil can help reduce inflammation and promote better nerve functioning.

Probiotics — Helps to restore or maintain a healthy symbiotic gut microbiota that decreases inflammation.

High potency multi-vitamin — Provides basic nutrients needed for immune function.

Digestive enzymes (1–2 capsules with meals) — May help with digestion and reduce autoimmune reactions to foods.

Vitamin B12 (1,000 micrograms daily) — Vitamin B12 helps with the formation of nerves.

Astaxanthin (2 milligrams, one to two times daily) — A powerful carotenoid antioxidant found in wild-caught salmon that can support the brain and nervous system. It can be found in certain fish oil supplements, helping to improve its effects.

According to research published by the MS Study Group of the TRIP-Graduate School at Goethe-University in Germany, certain "disease modifying nutricals" have also been shown to be helpful for managing multiple sclerosis. These nutricals include:

Green tea flavonoid extract (especially EGCG, or epigallocatechin-3-gallate), which has the ability to fight oxidative damage and supports metabolic health.

Curcumin, the active ingredient found in turmeric that has anti-inflammatory benefits and much more.

Mustard oil, which contains free radical-fighting glycosides.

Cannabis, which has analgesic and anti-spastic effects.

Use Essential Oils

Essential oils including frankincense oil and helichrysum oil naturally support the neurological system. In animal studies, frankincense has been shown to have many anti-inflammatory properties and to help support regeneration of damaged nerves and functional recovery. You may want to try frankincense oil as one of your multiple sclerosis natural treatments. Take 2 drops of frankincense internally three times a day for three weeks, then take one week off and repeat that cycle. You can also rub 2 drops of helichrysum oil on your temples and neck two times daily. Also, basil oil and cypress oil can improve circulation and muscular functions and therefore may help reduce MS symptoms.

Precautions

Symptoms of MS can be very similar to those caused by other diseases, so it's important to always get a proper diagnosis from a specialist. Visit a doctor if you notice changes such as unexplained loss of sensation, burning, pain and weakness. Children who are susceptible to MS should be given medical care right away, if possible. If you're concerned about how having MS will change your dietary or exercise needs, then consult with your doctor.

Foods to eat

Based on current and ongoing research, an MS-friendly diet should help people with MS manage their symptoms.

In particular, it should help manage disease progression and aim to minimize the effects that common MS symptoms have on overall quality of life.

Here is a list of foods to include on an MS-friendly diet:

- fruits and vegetables: all fresh fruits and vegetables
- grains: all grains, such as oats, rice, and quinoa
- nuts and seeds: all nuts and seeds
- fish: all fish, especially fresh fish and fatty oily fish, such as salmon and mackerel, as they're high in omega-3 fatty acids and vitamin D
- meats: all fresh meats, such as beef, chicken, lamb, and more, especially beef liver which is particularly high in vitamin D and biotin
- eggs: good source of biotin, vitamin D, and other important nutrients
- dairy products: such as milk, cheese, yogurt, and butter

- fats: healthy fats, such as olive, flaxseed, coconut, and avocado oils
- probiotic-rich foods: such as yogurt, kefir, sauerkraut, and kimchi
- beverages: water, herbal teas
- herbs and spices: all fresh herbs and spices

In short, the guidelines for an MS-friendly diet are similar to an overall nutrient-rich, well-balanced diet. However, it emphasizes consuming more plant-based foods and grains.

That is because plant-based foods and grains are higher in fiber, vitamins, minerals, and fluid, which can help with MS symptoms, such as constipation, fatigue, and bladder dysfunction.

They're also higher in plant-based compounds that function as antioxidants, which are molecules that help defend your cells against free radical damage and inflammation. These compounds may help fight inflammation and potentially slow MS progression.

Fish, particularly fatty fish, such as salmon and mackerel, appear to be beneficial for MS, possibly because they're high in anti-inflammatory omega-3 fatty acids. They're also high in vitamin D, which can help keep your bones strong when combined with calcium.

Current research on the effects of red meat and saturated fat intakes on MS symptoms shows mixed results. However, eating red meat in moderation, while focusing on more fruits, vegetables, and grains, is likely beneficial for people with MS.

Dairy products also show mixed results. In some studies, dairy products have been linked to disease activity. However, they're a good source of calcium, vitamin D, vitamin A, and potassium, so you can try including them in moderation on an MS-friendly diet. Talk with your doctor if you believe dairy products are making your MS symptoms worse.

In addition, some research shows that people with MS may have a higher risk of celiac disease, an autoimmune condition that causes damage to the small intestine in the presence of gluten.

Gluten is a group of proteins in wheat, barley, and rye.

If you have MS and experience extreme discomfort when eating gluten-based products, such as bread, pasta, crackers, and baked goods, it's important to notify your healthcare team to see whether you have celiac disease. Other symptoms of celiac disease include bloating, diarrhea, fatigue, abdominal pain, chronic headaches, and anemia.

People with MS who do not have celiac disease may still benefit from healthy grains in their diet.

Foods to avoid

While an MS-friendly diet allows plenty of nutrient-dense, delicious options, there are still some food groups you should limit to help manage MS symptoms.

- Most of these foods are linked to chronic inflammation. They include processed meats, refined carbs, trans fats, and sugar-sweetened beverages, just to name a few.
- Here's a list of foods to avoid if you have MS:
- processed meats: such as sausages, bacon, canned meats, and meats that are salted, smoked, or cured

- refined carbs: such as white bread, pasta, biscuits, and flour tortillas
- fried foods: such as french fries, fried chicken, mozzarella sticks, and doughnuts
- highly processed foods: such as fast food, potato chips, and convenience and frozen meals
- trans fats: such as margarine, shortening, and partially hydrogenated vegetable oils
- sugar-sweetened beverages: such as energy and sports drinks, soda, and sweet tea
- alcohol: limit consumption of all alcoholic beverages as much as possible

If you have celiac disease, aim to avoid all gluten-based foods, such as foods containing wheat, barley, and rye.

Specialty diets

Several diets specifically aim to help slow progression and prevent flare-ups of MS. They include the Swank diet and variations of the Wahls diet. These diets are popular within the community of individuals with MS.

The Swank diet for MS is a low-fat, low-saturated fat eating pattern that neurologist Dr. Roy Swank, MD, PhD, developed in 1948. Its recommendations include:

- avoid processed foods that contain saturated fat or hydrogenated oils
- limit saturated fat to 15 grams per day; consume no more than 20 to 50 grams per day of unsaturated fats
- avoid red meat for 1 year, then limit red meat to 3 ounces per week
- avoid dark meat poultry and limit fatty fish to 50 grams per day
- choose only dairy with 1% fat or less
- avoid egg yolks
- consume as many fruits and vegetables as you want
- enjoy whole grain breads, rice, and pastas
- snack on nuts and seeds daily
- consume 1 teaspoon of cod liver oil, and a multi-vitamin and mineral supplement daily

Research on the efficacy of the Swank diet is limited to a series of reports Dr. Swank published. The reports follow a group of individuals with RRMS who adhered to the Swank low fat diet for 50 years. Dr. Swank assessed individuals for compliance with the diet, frequency and severity of MS attacks, and performance status (wheelchair use, ability to walk, and ability to work).

Those who adhered to the diet (consumed 20 grams of fat or less) had fewer and less severe MS-related exacerbations than those who consumed greater than 20 grams of fat. Individuals with lower performance status at the start of the observation period or who were in the progressive phase of MS were likely to experience continued decline, even if they complied with the Swank diet.

While Swank's studies had a long follow-up duration and large cohort size, they were not randomized controlled trials and were subject to several forms of bias. Larger, better-designed studies are needed to determine whether the Swank diet can help improve symptoms or delay progression of MS.

Dr. Terry Wahls developed the modified Paleolithic Wahls diet for managing MS in 2008.

The Wahls diet is a version of the Paleolithic (Paleo) diet, which recommends you eat meat, fish, eggs, vegetables, fruits, nuts, seeds, herbs, spices, healthy fats, and oils, and that you avoid processed foods, sugar, grains, most dairy products, legumes, artificial sweeteners, vegetable oils, margarine, and trans fats.

The modified Paleo Wahls diet makes the following recommendations beyond the Paleo diet:

- eat nine or more cups of fruits and vegetables daily (three cups each of green leafy vegetables, sulfur-rich vegetables, and intensely colored fruits or vegetables)
- emphasize consumption of seaweed, algae, and nutritional yeast
- consume limited servings of gluten-free grains and legumes
- avoid eggs
- consume lower meat and fish intake than the Paleo diet

In one small randomized, controlled trial, 17 individuals with RRMS who followed the Wahls diet for three months experienced improved quality of life and less fatigue compared to those who continued their usual diet. More studies are needed to assess the effectiveness of the modified Paleo Wahls diet.

Dr. Wahls developed The Wahls Elimination diet in 2015, which recommends avoiding all grains (including those that are gluten-free), legumes, and nightshades (including tomatoes, white potatoes, eggplant, peppers, and seed spices) to reduce lectin in the diet.

It also recommends avoiding all dairy and allows for unlimited consumption of saturated fat. Like the modified Paleolithic Wahls diet, the Wahls Elimination diet recommends at least nine cups of fruits and vegetables daily, as well as seaweed, nutritional yeast, and fermented foods.

While a study comparing the impact of the Swank and Wahls Elimination diets on MS-related fatigue and quality of life is currently underway, no research is available on the efficacy of the Wahls Elimination diet.

It is important to note that diets that exclude whole food groups (like grains and dairy in the Wahls Elimination diet) increase the probability of nutritional insufficiency. However, taking supplements when on these diets can help reduce the risk of nutritional deficiency.

In addition to the diet guidelines above, people with MS may want to consider the following food tips to help manage their symptoms.

Make sure you eat enough food. Eating too few calories can cause fatigue.

Prep your meals in advance. If you have time, batch-making meals can help you save energy later. If you're often fatigued, this can be especially helpful.

Rearrange your kitchen. Place food, utensils, and other equipment in areas that are close by and easy for you to clean up. This will help you save energy.

Try "ready-to-use" items. Buying precut fruits and veggies can help you shave minutes off cooking time and make cooking simpler.

Make thicker drinks. If you have difficulty swallowing, preparing thicker beverages like a nutrient-rich smoothie may be easier to manage.

Soft foods may help. If chewing too much is making you fatigued, try choosing softer foods like baked fish, bananas, avocado, and cooked veggies.

Limit crumbly foods. If you have difficulty swallowing or find yourself choking on food often, consider limiting foods that crumble, such as toast and crackers.

Reach out for help. Even if you do not like asking for help, having members of your support network help with small tasks, like preparing meals, cleaning, or simply setting the table, can help ease your fatigue.

Stay active. Although exercise can make a person with MS feel fatigued, it's especially important for helping achieve and manage optimal health and a moderate weight. It's also important for preventing osteoporosis, which is more common among people with MS.

If you have other MS-related concerns not addressed above, it's important to notify your healthcare team. They can offer personalized tips to help you manage your symptoms better.

Following the Swank diet isn't about adhering to a strict meal plan but rather making food choices for meals and snacks that, over the course of a day, keep your total fat intake low. For example:

Breakfast

Fruit smoothie made with 1/4 cup each frozen raspberries, blueberries, and pineapple, half a frozen banana, and 1 cup of skim, soy, almond, or rice milk

One cup of coffee or tea, black or with a splash of non-dairy milk or cream

Morning snack

1 cup non-fat yogurt topped with berries and roasted walnuts

Lunch

Salad of dark leafy greens topped with one hard-boiled egg (one of three that are allowed during the course of a week), whatever mix of raw vegetables you enjoy (carrots, celery, cucumber, fennel, tomatoes), and 1/8 avocado

Whole grain crackers or a handful of baked tortilla chips

Afternoon snack

Almond-butter-and-sliced-apple sandwich on whole-grain bread

Dinner

4-ounce skinless breast

Vegetables (cauliflower, Brussels sprouts, broccoli, or a combination) tossed with olive oil and fresh herbs and roasted on a sheet pan

Brown rice

Optional: One glass of wine

Dessert

A slice of angel food cake

Chapter two

Multiple Sclerosis Diet Recipes
Great Green Salad

Yummy green feta salad, great for summer evenings! Add as many fruits and vegetables as you

Prep Time: 10 mins

Total Time: 10 mins

Servings: 4

Yield: 4 servings

Ingredients

4 tablespoons olive oil

2 tablespoons white wine vinegar

1 tablespoon Dijon mustard

½ teaspoon salt

½ teaspoon ground black pepper

1 pinch white sugar

1 teaspoon chopped fresh parsley

1 teaspoon fresh lemon juice

2 cloves garlic, chopped

1 avocados - peeled, pitted, and cubed

4 cups mixed salad greens

½ cup sliced almonds

2 ounces feta cheese, crumbled

Directions

In a large bowl, whisk together the olive oil, white wine vinegar, mustard, salt, pepper, sugar, parsley, lemon juice and garlic. Add the avocado, and stir to coat with the dressing.

Just before serving, add the salad greens, and toss to coat with dressing. Sprinkle sliced almonds and feta cheese over the top.

Nutrition Facts (per serving)

326 Calories 30g Fat 11g Carbs 7g Protein

Green Salad with Cranberry Vinaigrette

Green salad that is especially pretty to serve during the Christmas holidays.

Prep Time: 15 mins

Cook Time: 5 mins

Total Time: 20 mins

Servings: 8

Yield: 8 servings

Ingredients

1 cup sliced almonds

3 tablespoons red wine vinegar

⅓ cup olive oil

¼ cup fresh cranberries

1 tablespoon Dijon mustard

½ teaspoon minced garlic

½ teaspoon salt

½ teaspoon ground black pepper

2 tablespoons water

½ red onion, thinly sliced

4 ounces crumbled blue cheese

1 pound mixed salad greens

Directions

Preheat oven to 375 degrees F (190 degrees C). Arrange almonds in a single layer on a baking sheet. Toast in oven for 5 minutes, or until nuts begin to brown.

In a blender or food processor, combine the vinegar, oil, cranberries, mustard, garlic, salt, pepper, and water. Process until smooth.

In a large bowl, toss the almonds, onion, blue cheese, and greens with the vinegar mixture until evenly coated.

Nutrition Facts (per serving)

219 Calories 19g Fat 6g Carbs 7g Protein

Italian Leafy Green Salad

Grapeseed oil is the secret to this Italian greens salad. If you cannot find it, use olive oil.

Prep Time: 15 mins

Total Time: 15 mins

Servings: 6

Yield: 6 1-cup servings

Ingredients

2 cups romaine lettuce - torn, washed and dried

1 cup torn escarole

1 cup torn radicchio

1 cup torn red leaf lettuce

12 cherry tomatoes

½ red bell pepper, sliced into rings

½ green bell pepper, sliced in rings

¼ cup chopped green onions

Dressing:

¼ cup grapeseed oil

¼ cup balsamic vinegar

2 tablespoons lemon juice

2 tablespoons chopped fresh basil

salt and pepper to taste

Directions

Combine romaine, escarole, radicchio, red leaf lettuce, cherry tomatoes, bell peppers, and green onions in a large bowl.

Make dressing: Whisk together grapeseed oil, vinegar, lemon juice, basil, salt, and pepper in a small bowl.

Pour dressing over salad and toss well.

Nutrition Facts (per serving)

110 Calories 9g Fat 7g Carbs 1g Protein

Green Salad

This green salad is good for a side dish or a meal on its own. I make it often for my family and they always enjoy it.

Prep Time: 15 mins

Cook Time: 15 mins

Total Time: 30 mins

Servings: 8

Ingredients

½ cup chopped onion

½ cup chopped green bell pepper

2 (10 ounce) packages mixed salad greens

4 thinly sliced chicken deli meat, chopped

1 tomato, chopped

¼ teaspoon onion powder

3 dashes garlic powder

2 pinches salt and ground black pepper to taste

3 tablespoons balsamic vinaigrette salad dressing

Directions

Gather the ingredients.

Place onion and bell pepper in a microwave-safe bowl; heat in microwave on high until soft, about 1 to 2 minutes. Set aside to cool.

Combine onion, bell pepper, salad greens, deli meat, and tomato in a large salad bowl. Sprinkle with onion powder, garlic powder, salt, and black pepper; toss well to mix.

Pour on salad dressing; toss well and serve.

Enjoy!

Nutrition Facts (per serving)

47 Calories 2g Fat 5g Carbs 3g Protein

People tend to forget to eat salads and other raw foods in the cold winter weather. This salad is a good way to get your greens by combining somewhat heartier salad textures. I find that this salad is filling enough to be the main course, with a bit of bread or some rice cakes on the side. It will also work as an appetizer in a smaller serving.

Prep Time: 30 mins

Total Time: 30 mins

Servings: 4

Ingredients

Salad:

4 collard leaves, trimmed and finely chopped

⅓ bunch kale, trimmed and chopped

1 head romaine lettuce, chopped

¼ small head red cabbage, chopped

1 Bosc pear, cubed

½ Bermuda onion, finely diced

½ orange bell pepper, diced

½ Florida avocado - peeled, pitted, and diced

½ carrot, grated

5 cherry tomatoes, halved

7 walnut halves, crushed

2 tablespoons raisins, or to taste

Dressing:

6 tablespoons olive oil

3 tablespoons balsamic vinegar

1 tablespoon wildflower honey

1 tablespoon oregano, crushed

1 ½ teaspoons chili powder

1 teaspoon Dijon mustard

1 clove garlic, minced

½ teaspoon salt

¼ teaspoon crushed black peppercorns

Directions

Mix collard greens, kale, romaine, cabbage, pear, onion, orange bell pepper, avocado, carrot, tomatoes, walnuts, and raisins together in a large bowl.

Combine olive oil, vinegar, honey, oregano, chili powder, Dijon mustard, garlic, salt, and black pepper in a glass jar with a lid. Cover the jar with a lid and shake vigorously until dressing is well mixed. Pour dressing over salad; toss to coat.

Editor's Note:

Please note ingredient substitutions and serving size difference when using the magazine version of this recipe.

Nutrition Facts (per serving)

421 Calories 28g Fat 44g Carbs 8g Protein

Baked Tortilla Chips

Tasty tortilla chips baked at home with corn tortillas are much better than store-bought chips. With an amazing lime and cumin flavor, these crispy, golden chips taste great with your favorite salsa, guacamole, or hummus.

Prep Time: 10 mins

Cook Time: 15 mins

Total Time: 25 mins

Servings: 12

Ingredients

1 (12 ounce) package corn tortillas

3 tablespoons lime juice

1 tablespoon vegetable oil

1 teaspoon ground cumin

1 teaspoon chili powder

1 teaspoon salt

Directions

Gather all ingredients.

Preheat oven to 350 degrees F (175 degrees C).

Stack tortillas in layers of 5 or 6. Cut through each stack to make 8 wedges. Arrange wedges in a single layer on rimmed baking sheets.

Combine lime juice and oil in a spray bottle or mister; shake until well mixed. Spray the tops of the tortilla wedges until slightly moist.

Combine cumin, chili powder, and salt in a small bowl; sprinkle mixture over the chips.

Bake in the preheated oven for 7 minutes.

Remove from the oven. Flip chips, then mist and season again.

Return to the oven, rotating the pans and switching racks. Bake, checking often to ensure they don't burn, until chips are lightly browned and crisp, 5 to 8 more minutes.

Remove from the oven and cool slightly before serving. Chips will crisp up more as they cool.

Enjoy with a side of salsa!

Recipe Tip

Even stale or dried-out corn tortillas will give good results in this recipe.

Nutrition Facts (per serving)

74 Calories 2g Fat 13g Carbs 2g Protein

Homemade Baked Tortilla Chips

Homemade baked tortilla chips that are very easy to make.

Prep Time: 5 mins

Cook Time: 5 mins

Total Time: 10 mins

Servings: 10

Yield: 10 servings

Ingredients

1 (12 ounce) package flour tortillas

1 drizzle olive oil

1 pinch salt to taste

Directions

Preheat the oven to 350 degrees F (175 degrees C).

Cut tortillas into 6 wedges each. Place on a baking sheet and drizzle with olive oil. Season with salt.

Bake in the preheated oven until golden and crisp, about 5 minutes.

Nutrition Facts (per serving)

115 Calories 3g Fat 19g Carbs 3g Protein

Use this corn chip recipe for a batch of fried or baked tortilla chips that are lightly seasoned with salt.

Prep Time: 10 mins

Cook Time: 25 mins

Total Time: 35 mins

Servings: 12

Yield: 72 chips

Ingredients

1 cup oil for frying, or as needed

12 (6 inch) corn tortillas, cut into 6 wedges each

salt to taste

Directions

Heat 1/4 inch oil in a large, heavy saucepan to 375 degrees F (190 degrees C).

Working in small batches, fry tortilla wedges in hot oil until crisp, about 2 minutes. Remove from the heat and drain on paper towels. Season warm chips with salt.

Tips

The chips can be baked in an oven preheated to 350 degrees F (175 degrees C) until crisp, about 5 minutes.

Editor's Note

We have determined the nutritional value of oil for frying based on a retention value of 10% after cooking. The exact amount may vary depending on cook time and temperature, ingredient density, and the specific type of oil used.

Nutrition Facts (per serving)

162 Calories

18g Fat

Praline Cinnamon Tortilla Chips

Chips made from flour tortillas which have been dipped in canola oil and then in a cinnamon-sugar mix and baked. They come out tasting like really crisp praline cinnamon chips.

Prep Time: 15 mins

Cook Time: 5 mins

Additional Time: 15 mins

Total Time: 35 mins

Servings: 4

Yield: 4 servings

Ingredients

1 cup white sugar

1 teaspoon ground cinnamon

½ teaspoon chili powder

⅛ teaspoon ground black pepper, or more to taste

½ cup canola oil

1 (8 ounce) package flour tortillas, cut into 2-inch squares

Directions

Stir sugar, cinnamon, chili powder, and black pepper in a shallow bowl until thoroughly combined.

Pour canola oil into a separate bowl.

Set an oven rack about 6 inches from the heat source and preheat the oven's broiler.

Dip tortilla squares into canola oil on both sides and press into the seasoned sugar mixture; arrange coated chips on baking sheets.

Broil chips until sugar bubbles and chips are crisp, about 2 minutes; watch carefully to prevent burning. Turn the chips over and broil other sides until browned, another 2 minutes. Let cool before serving.

Cook's Notes:

Use canola oil. Do not use vegetable oil or olive oil.

The thicker the sugar mixture is on each rectangle, the darker, crunchier and quicker to burn each will be. For this reason, sometimes I sprinkle it on rather than dip, but it depends on my mood more than anything.

Editor's Note:

We have determined the nutritional value of canola oil for cooking based on a retention value of 10%. The exact amount will vary depending on cooking time, exact temperature, and ingredient density, among other factors.

Nutrition Facts (per serving)

397 Calories 7g Fat 80g Carbs 5g Protein

Use up that leftover brown rice and try something new for breakfast. Experiment with it to make it your own, you can try using any mixture of dried fruit instead of the blueberries.

Prep Time: 5 mins

Cook Time: 25 mins

Total Time: 30 mins

Servings: 2

Yield: 2 servings

Ingredients

1 cup cooked brown rice

1 cup 2% low-fat milk

2 tablespoons dried blueberries

1 dash cinnamon

1 tablespoon honey

1 egg

¼ teaspoon vanilla extract

1 tablespoon butter

Directions

Combine the cooked brown rice, milk, blueberries, cinnamon, and honey in a small saucepan. Bring to a boil, then reduce heat to low and simmer for 20 minutes.

Beat the egg in a small bowl. Temper the egg by whisking in some of the hot rice, a tablespoon at a time until you have incorporated about 6 tablespoons. Stir the egg into the rice along with the vanilla and butter, and continue cooking over low heat for 1 to 2 minutes to thicken.

Nutrition Facts (per serving)

318 Calories 12g Fat 45g Carbs 10g Protein

Easy Oven Brown Rice

I am a terrible rice cook, but once I tried this method I can be confident that it will turn out every time!

Prep Time: 10 mins

Cook Time: 1 hr

Total Time: 1 hr 10 mins

Servings: 6

Yield: 3 cups

Ingredients

1 ½ cups brown rice

1 teaspoon salt

2 tablespoons butter

3 cups boiling water

Directions

Preheat oven to 400 degrees F (200 degrees C).

Place rice, salt, and butter in a casserole dish that has a cover. Pour boiling water over rice; stir.

Cover and bake in preheated oven until liquid is absorbed and rice is tender, about 1 hour. Remove from oven, fluff with fork, and serve hot.

Recipe Tip

This recipe can be scaled, but the cook time may need to be adjusted accordingly.

Nutrition Facts (per serving)

206 Calories 5g Fat 36g Carbs 4g Protein

This is comfort food at its best with mild flavors and it's simple to make. This is a very versatile dish: if you prefer, you can use almonds in place of the cashews, and cilantro in place of the parsley.

Servings: 4

Yield: 4 servings

Ingredients

1 ½ cups water

½ teaspoon salt

¾ cup uncooked brown rice

3 tablespoons butter

1 ½ cups chopped onion

1 clove garlic, minced

2 carrots, sliced

2 cups fresh sliced mushrooms

1 cup chickpeas

2 eggs, beaten

freshly ground black pepper

¼ cup chopped fresh parsley

¼ cup chopped cashews

Directions

Bring 1-1/2 cups water to boil, add rice. Bring contents back to a boil, cover the pot and simmer for 45-50 minutes, or until rice is tender.

Approximately 20 minutes before rice is finished cooking heat the butter in a large skillet over medium heat. Stir in onions and saute them, stirring frequently until they soften. Add the garlic and carrots and continue stirring for 5 minutes.

Place mushrooms inside of skillet and cook until mushrooms begin to brown, about 10 minutes. Add the chickpeas and cook 1 more minute.

When the rice is finished cooking pour the eggs into the skillet and cook the mixture, stirring constantly until the eggs are cooked. Remove the skillet from the heat, stir in pepper, parsley, and nuts.

Spoon the cooked rice into the skillet and stir well. Serve the pilaf hot with soy sauce on the side for added flavor.

Nutrition Facts (per serving)

409 Calories 17g Fat 54g Carbs 13g Protein

Lemony Shrimp over Brown Rice

This shrimp dish was something I threw together one night and my family loved it. It's really easy, healthy, and tasty!

Prep Time: 15 mins

Cook Time: 20 mins

Total Time: 35 mins

Servings: 4

Yield: 4 servings

Ingredients

1 cup brown rice

1 ⅔ cups water

3 tablespoons butter

3 tablespoons olive oil

2 cloves garlic, minced

½ cup white wine

2 tablespoons fresh lemon juice

1 ½ pounds medium shrimp - peeled and deveined

¼ cup chopped fresh flat-leaf parsley

½ teaspoon cornstarch

Directions

Combine the brown rice and water in a small saucepan. Bring to a boil, reduce heat to low and cook until all the water is absorbed, about 25 minutes.

Melt the butter with the olive oil in a skillet over medium heat; cook the garlic in the butter and oil until fragrant, 1 to 2 minutes. Pour in the wine and lemon juice; reduce heat to medium-low and simmer. Stir in the shrimp and cook until the shrimp turns pink, stirring regularly, 5 to 7 minutes. Sprinkle the parsley over the shrimp and cook another 2 minutes. Add the cornstarch to the liquid and stir until it thickens, about 1 minute more. Serve hot over the brown rice.

Nutrition Facts (per serving)

551 Calories 23g Fat 40g Carbs 39g Protein

Garlic Chicken Fried Brown Rice

Leftover brown rice is reborn in this chicken fried rice with peppers and onions. Black pepper, paprika, or dried parsley may be used to season after this is cooked.

Prep Time: 20 mins

Cook Time: 15 mins

Total Time: 35 mins

Servings: 3

Yield: 3 servings

Ingredients

2 tablespoons vegetable oil, divided

8 ounces skinless, boneless chicken breast, cut into strips

½ red bell pepper, chopped

½ cup green onion, chopped

4 cloves garlic, minced

3 cups cooked brown rice

2 tablespoons light soy sauce

1 tablespoon rice vinegar

1 cup frozen peas, thawed

Directions

Heat 1 tablespoon of vegetable oil in a large skillet set over medium heat. Add the chicken, bell pepper, green onion and garlic. Cook and stir until the chicken is cooked through, about 5 minutes. Remove the chicken to a plate and keep warm.

Heat the remaining tablespoon of oil in the same skillet over medium-high heat. Add the rice; cook and stir to heat through. Stir in the soy sauce, rice vinegar and peas, and continue to cook for 1 minute. Return the chicken mixture to the skillet and stir to blend with the rice and heat through before serving.

Nutrition Facts (per serving)

444 Calories 13g Fat 57g Carbs 24g Protein

Easy enough for people who can't make rice at all, and everyone will love it!

Prep Time: 5 mins

Cook Time: 1 hr

Total Time: 1 hr 5 mins

Servings: 4

Yield: 4 to 6 servings

Ingredients

1 ½ cups uncooked long-grain white rice

1 (14 ounce) can beef broth

1 (10.5 ounce) can condensed French onion soup

¼ cup butter, melted

1 tablespoon Worcestershire sauce

1 tablespoon dried basil leaves

Directions

Preheat oven to 350 degrees F (175 degrees C).

In a 2 quart casserole dish combine rice, broth, soup, butter, Worcestershire sauce and basil.

Bake covered for 1 hour, stirring once after 30 minutes.

Nutrition Facts (per serving)

425 Calories 14g Fat 66g Carbs 9g Protein

Perfect Hard-Boiled Eggs

Use this recipe for perfectly cooked hard-boiled eggs. By adding a little vinegar and salt, the eggshell peels off so easily without tearing or sticking. I have been making them this way for years!

Prep Time: 5 mins

Cook Time: 20 mins

Additional Time: 15 mins

Total Time: 40 mins

Servings: 8

Yield: 8 hard-boiled eggs

Ingredients

1 tablespoon salt

¼ cup distilled white vinegar

6 cups water

8 large eggs

Directions

Gather all ingredients.

Combine salt, vinegar, and water in a large pot, and bring to a boil over high heat.

Add eggs one at a time, being careful not to crack them. Reduce the heat to a gentle boil, and cook for 14 minutes.

Once eggs have cooked, remove them from the hot water, and place into a container of ice water or cold, running water. Cool completely, about 15 minutes. Store in the refrigerator up to 1 week.

Enjoy!

Nutrition Facts (per serving)

72 Calories 5g Fat 0g Carbs 6g Protein

Pressure Cooker Hard-Boiled Eggs

Pressure cooker hard-boiled eggs aren't any quicker to make (the pressure cooker's usual claim to fame), but here's why it's great: it actually makes fresh eggs easy to peel! If you happen to raise chickens or have access to really fresh eggs, a pressure cooker is the best way to make hard-cooked eggs.

Prep Time: 5 mins

Cook Time: 6 mins

Additional Time: 35 mins

Total Time: 46 mins

Servings: 8

Ingredients

2 cups water, or as needed

8 fresh eggs

4 cups cold water

4 cups ice cubes

Directions

Fill a pressure cooker with the minimum amount of water specified by the manufacturer. Place eggs in the steamer basket above the water. Seal the lid and bring the pressure cooker up to low pressure.

Cook, maintaining low pressure, for 6 minutes. Remove the pressure cooker from heat and allow the pressure to drop for 5 minutes.

Combine cold water and ice in a large bowl.

Use the quick-release method to open the pressure cooker. Transfer hot eggs to ice water using an oven mitt or spoon. Cool completely, about 30 minutes.

Recipe Tip

Letting the pressure cooker reach high pressure will cause eggs to crack.

Nutrition Facts (per serving)

63 Calories 4g Fat 0g Carbs 6g Protein

Divine Hard-Boiled Eggs

The method in this recipe hard boils eggs perfectly every time without turning the yolks green. It also includes the best method for easy peeling!

Prep Time: 5 mins

Cook Time: 15 mins

Additional Time: 2 hrs 30 mins

Total Time: 2 hrs 50 mins

Servings 12

Yield: 12 hard-boiled eggs

Ingredients

12 large eggs

Directions

Place eggs in a pot; pour enough water over the eggs to cover. Cover the pot and bring to a boil over high heat.

Remove pot from the heat; let sit, covered, for 15 minutes.

Fill a large bowl halfway with cold water; transfer eggs into cold water. Replace the water with cold water as needed to keep cold until eggs are completely cooled. Chill eggs in refrigerator for at least 2 hours before peeling.

Nutrition Facts (per serving)

72 Calories 5g Fat 0g Carbs 6g Protein

Steam eggs in a steamer basket for the easiest way to make hard-cooked eggs. Look no further for a foolproof method — fresh or old, they are always perfectly cooked and easy to peel.

Prep Time: 5 mins

Cook Time: 15 mins

Additional Time: 20 mins

Total Time: 40 mins

Servings: 12

Yield: 12 eggs

Ingredients

12 eggs, at room temperature

Directions

Place a steamer insert into a pot and fill with water to just below the bottom of the steamer. Bring water to just below a boil over medium heat. Gently place the eggs in the steamer insert, cover the pot, and steam for 15 minutes.

Immediately transfer eggs to a bowl of ice water until cool enough to handle. Make a small crack on the large end of each egg and place eggs back into the ice water for about 20 minutes, then peel.

Nutrition Facts (per serving)

72 Calories 5g Fat 0g Carbs 6g Protein

Hard-Boiled Egg Sandwich

These are so good! I have been making these hard-boiled egg sandwiches for years and we absolutely LOVE them. This is a great on-the-go breakfast or just a different way to use up leftover hard-boiled eggs. Enjoy!

Prep Time: 10 mins

Total Time: 10 mins

Servings: 1

Yield: 1 sandwich

Ingredients

2 slices white bread, toasted

1 tablespoon butter, softened

2 tablespoons whipped cream cheese

1 hard-boiled egg, sliced

5 dashes hot pepper sauce (such as Frank's RedHot®), or to taste

1 pinch salt and ground black pepper to taste

Directions

Butter each slice of toast. Spread 1 tablespoon cream cheese onto each slice.

Layer hard-boiled egg slices evenly onto 1 slice of toast. Add hot sauce, salt, and pepper. Top with other slice of toast.

Recipe Tip

You can substitute your favorite bread for white bread if you prefer.

Nutrition Facts (per serving)

372 Calories 24g Fat 27g Carbs 11g Protein

Basic Fruit Smoothie

This is a great fruit smoothie recipe consisting of fruit, fruit juice, and ice. I like to use whatever fresh fruits I crave that day... Berries, mangos, papayas, kiwi fruit, etc. Experiment with your favorites!

Prep Time: 10 mins

Total Time: 10 mins

Servings: 4

Ingredients

1 quart strawberries, hulled

2 fresh peaches - peeled, pitted, and sliced

1 banana, broken into chunks

2 cups ice

1 cup orange-peach-mango juice

Directions

Gather all ingredients.

Combine strawberries, peaches, and banana in a blender; blend until smooth.

Add ice and pour in juice; blend again to desired consistency.

Enjoy!

Nutrition Facts (per serving)

118 Calories 1g Fat 29g Carbs 2g Protein

This is a great smoothie for breakfast - and sometimes dinner! You can substitute the orange juice with any mix of juices or even soy milk! The soy milk adds more of a milk shake quality than the juice does.

Prep Time: 5 mins

Total Time: 5 mins

Servings: 5

Yield: 4 to 6 drinks

Ingredients

2 frozen bananas, skins removed and cut in chunks

½ cup frozen blueberries

1 cup orange juice

1 tablespoon honey (Optional)

1 teaspoon vanilla extract (Optional)

Directions

Place bananas, blueberries and juice in a blender, puree. Use honey and/or vanilla to taste. Use more or less liquid depending on the thickness you want for your smoothie.

Nutrition Facts (per serving)

88 Calories 0g Fat 21g Carbs 1g Protein

Fruit and Yogurt Smoothie

This yogurt smoothie recipe is delicious! You may substitute the strawberries for any other berries or fruit.

Prep Time: 5 mins

Total Time: 5 mins

Servings: 2

Ingredients

1 cup strawberries

1 banana

½ cup yogurt

¼ cup pineapple juice

1 ½ teaspoons white sugar

1 teaspoon orange juice

1 teaspoon milk

Directions

Gather all ingredients.

Combine strawberries, banana, yogurt, pineapple juice, sugar, orange juice, and milk in a blender.

Blend until smooth.

Nutrition Facts (per serving)

146 Calories 1g Fat 31g Carbs 5g Protein

Conclusion

Healthy dietary choices can benefit people with MS by boosting overall well-being and quality of life. Certain dietary habits may change the condition's progression or prevent specific symptoms or complications, such as cardiovascular disease.

A range of special diets may help manage MS symptoms and reduce the chance of complications. However, more research is necessary to assess the effectiveness of these diets, and a person should consult a doctor before making any major dietary changes.

People with MS may wish to avoid highly processed foods, saturated fats, and added salt and sugar. Minimally processed whole foods, such as fruits, vegetables, pulses, legumes, and oily fish, are better choices.